MANIC DEPRESSIVE PSYCHOSIS THROUGH THE EYES OF THE BEHOLDER

MANIC DEPRESSIVE PSYCHOSIS THROUGH THE EYES OF THE BEHOLDER

Priscilla Sendelbach

iUniverse, Inc.

New York Lincoln Shanghai

MANIC DEPRESSIVE PSYCHOSIS THROUGH THE EYES OF THE BEHOLDER

iUniverse books may be ordered through booksellers or by contacting:

iUniverse
2021 Pine Lake Road, Suite 100
Lincoln, NE 68512
www.iuniverse.com
1-800-Authors (1-800-288-4677)

ISBN-13: 978-0-595-38285-9 (pbk)
ISBN-13: 978-0-595-82656-8 (ebk)
ISBN-10: 0-595-38285-1 (pbk)
ISBN-10: 0-595-82656-3 (ebk)

Printed in the United States of America

To: Christina Kloker Young,

You gave me the inspiration to write this. This is my past, but because of your help my future looks a lot brighter.

All my love, Priscilla

Contents

Acknowledgement

Prisicilla Sendelbach has been a gift sent to me soon after I accepted the job of Executive Director of the Mental Health Association of Summit County, of Ohio in 1979. My education was in Elementary education, music, business and counseling, but I was not prepared to understand the world that people who have serious mental health issues experience until Priscilla became my teacher. In Japan, the word for teacher is sensei and they are highly respected and revered. In Japan people bow in a special way to teachers. I would gladly bow to her as I respect her and I am humbled by Priscilla. I feel so blessed to have had Priscilla come into my life as she made my advocacy efforts strong persistent and effective. She has taught me about the pain and suffering that depression brings into peoples lives and the behaviors that are often uncontrollable. She and her dear husband Michael became my teachers and helped me understand the need for a first class system of care for the patient and their families. She has courage and has survived so many difficuties that came her way because of her diagnosis. This courage not to give into the pain and stigma was a great example to me to stand before political and public groups and teach the needs of the patients and their families. When the fundraising part of the job became so difficult in the community it was Priscilla and Mike that went out to ask for help and stood beside me as I planned activities. During a bike-a-thon, they rode their bikes with Dr. Mosteller and my daughter. Rev. Lisa Wolfe. They stood at the shopping center to collect signatures for legislation and answered some difficult questions from the public. The work of advocating for those who sometimes can't speak for themselves is of overwhelming and there is a wish at times to give up. But Priscilla was always an inspiration as she never gave up on her difficulties and accepted her challenge.

She and Michael have taught me about patience and love as they are an amazing example of profound love for their family and each other. She has also taught me about truth as she is a woman who always tells the truth. She is also one of the most caring people for the needs of others I have ever known. She is now serving her church as a volunteer and continues to care for her children and grandchildren and family. It was rare that Priscilla asked me "why did this happen to me?" She accepted her situation, was grateful to those around her who supported her and sympathetic for those who were not as fortunate as she. I am awed by her positive attitude and ability to face the realities of her situation and find a solution. We all have a limited time in life to do the work we feel is our reason for being. Priscilla has accepted a difficult situation and become a great teacher. I will always give her credit for inspiring and teaching me to become the best advocate for those with mental health difficulties I could be. She gave me courage and information to testify before public policy bodies, tour mental health facilities, and speak out loud and clear to the press. It was Priscilla's words of wanting to find a "cure" for this terrible disability that helped me fundraise and ask for improved services. Her faith in her God, her family, her church and herself is an inspiration.

With deep respect for my friend, Priscilla,
Christina Kloker Young November, 2005

Special Thanks to Rudy Libertini, Executive Director of The Mental Health Association of Summit County, Inc., for all of his assistance in helping me to write and develop my story.

Introduction

Many years ago, there was a very special person in my life. I was quite young at that time, and, I really didn't understand why he kept going in and out of the hospital. I knew he was in a lot of pain. Not only was he in pain physically, but emotionally he was hurting badly. He had his ups and downs, and, finally he passed away. He died from cancer.

Every year I would visit his grave, but, this year was different. Emotionally devastated, severely depressed and having just been released from the hospital with a diagnosis of Manic Depressive Psychosis, I went to the cemetery. I put a beautiful wreath on his grave, and, as I bent down to brush off the leaves, I spoke to him "You probably know I have an illness, too. It is not a physical illness like you had, and, I don't have the physical pain you suffered, but, I have emotional pain. The same kind of emotional pain you suffered learning of your illness. You had your ups and downs, and, you were in and out of the hospital continually. Your family understood your illness and coped with it the best they could. My family has trouble understanding my illness because it is emotional and bewildering to them."

A lot of families of mentally ill patients just don't understand how or why it happens. It's quite sad because the information is readily available. They are scared and just don't seem to read it.

I continued, "You had cancer and eventually died after a two year struggle. The mentally ill also struggle with life. Sometimes it seems hopeless and they commit suicide to be free from their own emotional pain. Let me tell you something. Your family loved you and was always there for you when you needed them. They supported you and they were with you every step of the way. I wish my family and friends would try to understand my illness because I need their support so desperately. I cannot understand why they won't reach out. After all, your family and my family were one and the same. You see, I am your sister."

MANIC DEPRESSIVE PSYCHOSIS A PERSONAL PERSPECTIVE

I cannot speak on this subject from a licensed psychiatrist's or psychologist's point of view, but, I will try to explain it from my point of view—the patient.

When I am in the manic state of the illness, I cannot be slowed down. I have the ability to manipulate some people. My mind races to the point where my thoughts run together. When I am manic, I feel great. I come up with all sorts of exciting projects and need little or no sleep. My manic state appears suddenly and, when gone untreated may last anywhere from a few hours to days, weeks, or even months. When anyone tries to put a damper on this feeling of great elation, I become erratic and sometimes I end up in an explosive state.

I also suffer from severe to mild depression-the other side of my illness. Depression, I feel is the most devastating part of my illness. If the depression is mild, I tend to withdraw from my family. Feelings of anxiety overcome my body, and I feel like an absolute failure. During the past eight years I have on two occasions become suicidal.

Manic Depression Psychosis is a bipolar disorder. My psychiatrist and psychologist both agree that I tend to be more on the manic side of the illness. Usually I will get manic and come back to a mild high. I feel fortunate that I don't suffer from the attacks of depression. I do, quite frequently, have severe waves of depression that ravage my body. To be quite honest, when they hit me without warning, I am prone to suicidal thoughts.

Stress plays an important part. When under extreme stress, I notice I experience more mood swings then normal. I am quite vulnerable to stress, and, I tend to be subject to erratic and explosive episodes when it starts to mount. Over the years, I have gradually established an equilibrium. But, when the stress begins to mount, I know I am in need of medical attention. It hasn't been easy for me to live with my mood swings, but, then again, it hasn't been easy for my family and friends either. On several occasions, my behavior was so unstable that it led to psychiatric hospitalization.

I feel fortunate that I have private insurance. In conjunction with my husband's benefits, we can afford the best psychiatric care available. I feel that mental illness should be treated as any other illness. Our insurance covers 50%. However, some hospitalization plans do not cover any mental health problems. There are a lot of people suffering needlessly. There is help available through the public mental health system. People, who aren't as fortunate as I am to have private insurance, can get the help they need by contacting their local Mental Health Association in the area in which they reside.

When you or your family feel defeated by mental illnes remember, you must have faith and a strong belief in God. If your family falls short of the support you so desperately need, remember this, "You are not alone." It was very devastating being rejected by my family because I suffer from a mental illness. I lost the love of my sisters and my father and, in the past, have been quite bitter. Once I was so torn that I talked to a priest. He told me that when a problem is just too much for me to handle, put it in God's hands and he will take care of it.

1

I was born third of four children. I was two months shy of being seven when my brother died of cancer at the age of fourteen. Having been very close to him, this was a very traumatic experience for me. When told of his death, I went into a rage. I insisted he be buried in the front yard so that I could be close to him. I believe my parents, being so grief stricken themselves, didn't recognize the grief I was experiencing. I don't blame them for their reaction. In my heart I now believe they could not handle my brother's death. How were they going to help me deal with it?

I can remember the funeral as if it were yesterday. I remember going to the funeral home and standing by his casket in disbelief. The more I stared, the more it looked as though he were breathing. I cried and cried telling my father that he wasn't dead, that he was truly alive. To put me out of my emotional state, my father, not knowing how to calm me down, lashed out and smacked me in the mouth. When we went to the graveside where he was to be buried, I refused to leave. A big crane came forward to lift the casket into the ground and I cried and cried, trying to explain to my father that my brother was alive. Once again, my father lashed out and smacked me. I was never able or given the chance, to talk about my emotions. My grief was silenced due to the threat of being smacked again. Life does go on after death, but, I know a part of me died with my brother. I was like his shadow and in his passing I was filled with anger and hate. I was now to become the middle child.

My father was grief stricken. He felt that if there were truly a God, he wouldn't have taken away his only son. On Sundays, he told us children that if we didn't want to attend church with our mother that, as far as he was concerned, we didn't have to go. He also didn't believe in doctors. My mother's thoughts and feelings were completely different.

Looking back on my childhood, I can remember, even through my teens, that every time I would get 'out of hand' my father would lash out and hit me. I can even remember times when my mother would try and pull him off me, screaming at him that he didn't know his own strength and that he was going to hurt me. When push came to shove and nothing seemed to work, I would tell him, "Go ahead! Hit me again if it makes you feel better." He would go into a rage pick me up, and proceed to the bathroom. My father was a strong person. He would place me, fighting and kicking, clothes and all under the shower, turn on the cold water and say, "This will cool you off." Looking back, I think I took more showers with my clothes than I did with them off.

At the dinner table, if I didn't like what was being serve and wouldn't eat, he would go into a rage. He would make me sit and sit until he was convinced I wasn't going to eat. Then he would tackle me to the floor and force cod liver oil down my throat.

My mother, on the other hand, never let us go to bed hungry, Sometimes she would come into my room at night with something to eat. She always said that each of us girls were different, but she loved us all the same.

Being the middle child, my father was always comparing me with my two sisters. I felt a need to please my father and to compete with my sisters. Being very outgoing and athletically inclined I took the place of the son that he had lost. We became 'buddies'. It was my only means of competing with my two sisters for his love.

During my school years, I never achieved high marks academically, but, I was a high achiever when it came to sports. Much to my father's delight, I excelled in baseball, basketball, volleyball and golf. However, my antics during school were quite stressful to mother. On more than one occasion, she was summoned to the school to act as liaison.

Being my dad's 'buddy,' I now got anything I wanted. At the age of 16, my father bought me my first motorcycle. My mother was beside herself. She begged him to return it, fearing I would get hurt. Much to my mother's dismay, I kept it. My dad even went out and bought me a car. So at the age of 16, I had my own car and motorcycle. I began smoking and drinking. My father, of course thought this was funny. Needless to say, my mother's feeling were quite the opposite. Upon graduation, one dubious honor was bestowed upon me. In my senior year, due to my behavior, I was voted "Class Clown"

Upon graduation, it was time to look for a job. To please father, I applied, and was accepted, at the same major rubber company he was employed by. At the same time, I was also accepted by another rubber company in the area. My decision, of course, was to work where my father was employed. To say the least, he was really delighted. My antic behavior followed me right into work. My father thought anything I did was funny. At work, the main topic of conversation between him and friends would be me. I had set out to get his attention, and that is exactly what I had achieved. The only reason I was able to hold down a job was the fact that I was good at what I did, and I knew it. During my employment, especially the first three years, my desk was moved on numerous occasions. I was even sent to the Personnel Department concerning my attitude and behavior.

At the age of 21, I started drinking quite heavily and got involved in drugs. My parents had no idea I was on drugs. While at work one day, I became quite sick and was taken to the plant hospital. Of course, they could find nothing wrong. I became quite ill and started throwing up blood. After being examined by a doctor, I was informed that I was pregnant. How was I going tell my father and mother? I did tell them, and my father informed me I was getting married immediately and having the baby. I tried to explain to him that under no circumstances would I have this child, due to drugs I was on. I just knew he was going lash out and hit me. The look in my father's eyes was frightening. He told me I had hurt him badly, and, that I was a complete failure as human being. He even asked how he could have raised a child that turned out this way. He told my mom, let's go to the golf course, if I'm lucky I will get hit in the head by a golf ball.

I had already made plans to go to New York where it was legal to have an abortion. I didn't believe in abortion, but, with my drug problem, I really felt I had no alternative. Reluctantly, my father drove me to the airport. I had the abortion returning home the same day. Against doctors' orders I had signed myself out of the hospital right after the procedure. I was warned that, in doing so, the hospital would not be responsible if I started to hemorrhage.

Emotionally, the abortion took its toll on me. All I knew was I had killed a human being, and, I didn't care if I bled to death. Death would have been easier than facing my father again. My mother came into my room upon my return. Her main concern was how I felt. She worried so about me. I told her I had signed myself out against doctors orders and she begged me to see a doctor here in town to make sure I was alright. I did see a doctor and I was fine physically. But, my mother knew I wasn't fine emotionally.

At this point in my life, I know I had failed my father and I started drinking even more. I got another job tending bar here in town, so, I was hardly ever home. I didn't want to go home. I would work all day and all night because I didn't want to see that look on his face. The emotional pain I went through was traumatic. I hadn't wanted the abortion and felt as though I'd committed murder. It was a heavy burden for me to carry and, when I look back on it, a feeling of tremendous sadness overwhelms me.

2

At the age of 23, I got married on a whim. I didn't love this man, but, my father was putting pressure on me to settle down and make something of my life. A life he felt was in ruins. Even though I was put under pressure my parents didn't think I should marry Kenneth. The marriage lasted two weeks. Upon my return home after this whirlwind affair, my father was totally embarrassed. Again, in his eyes, I had failed.

Still on drugs and running wild, I met my present husband. He went to school with me, but, he was so shy and quiet, I never paid any attention to him at first. We were as different as night and day. In fact, the night I did sit down and talk with him, I was preparing leave on vacation with friends the next day. Upon my return two weeks later, Michael phoned and asked me out. He didn't do drugs and he only had an occasional drink. He was a devout Catholic he led a completely different lifestyle than I did. Things began change for me. Before I knew it, I was going to church. I drank on occasion, but, drugs were definitely out of my life.

My mother and father both liked Michael. In fact, the only complaint my father voiced was that Michael was Catholic. After a year of dating, Michael asked me to marry him. This posed a big problem since, having been divorced, the Catholic church still recognized my first marriage. For Michael and I to be married in his church, which he felt strongly about, they would need to grant me a dispensation. If granted, it would make my first marriage null and void, and, I would be permitted to marry Michael in his church. The dispensation was only part of my problem. I truly loved Michael, but, in my heart, I knew I would have to tell him about the abortion. I also knew how strongly he felt about the issue. His reaction to the news was that he personally did not believe in abortion but, that God was forgiving and my past was my past. He also wanted me to try to forgive myself. The dispensation came through and our wedding took place. Michael was delighted. I really took an interest in the church, wanting more and more knowledge about its teachings. Baptized Lutheran, a religion I knew nothing about, I talked to a priest and began religious instructions, much to my father's dismay. Before my conversion to Catholicism, it was required that I go to confession. I had a hard time with this because, as I explained to Michael, I could not, in good faith, become Catholic unless I told the priest about the abortion. In confession, I explained to the priest my past, and he asked me if there was anything else I would like to add. My heart went into my stomach. I managed to tell him of the abortion. He said, and I will never forget it, "God is all good and forgiving, but, you my child, must learn to forgive yourself." I needed religion in my life, and, if I was going to have children I wanted to have religion in theirs.

Michael and I were married on June 1, 1974. It was our intention to wait at least two years before we had children. But, plans don't always work out the way you want them to.

It was July of 1974, when I became ill to the point of being rushed into the emergency room. The doctor on call did some blood work. When the results came back, he told me, Michael, and my mother that I was suffering from a vitamin deficiency. I was two weeks pregnant. Michael was ecstatic, even though we hadn't planned on children so soon. I was quite upset and afraid throughout entire pregnancy that something would go wrong, or maybe, due to my past drug problem the child would not be normal and healthy. The only thing that worried my mother was the fact she didn't feel I was ready to take care of a child. Much to our delight, our first son was born March 5, 1975.

During this time, my parents had moved to Florida. We were living in their house, watching over it. My mother didn't want to sell it until she was absolutely sure they wanted to live there. When they decided to make Florida their permanent home, they offered the house to Michael. I desperately needed this house, because I always felt my brother's presence here. We bought the house. Upon their arrival to sign the needed papers, Michael, my parents, and I sat down to dinner. My dad started smarting off to me and I smarted off back. Michael immediately spoke up, much to my mother's surprise, and said "She is my wife. She may be your daughter, but, I don't like you talking to her that way." The look on my father's face was pure astonishment. None of his sons-in-law had ever spoken up like Michael had done. I actually thought, in the back of my mind, that he was going to lash out at Michael, but, he didn't say a word. All my mother could do was clap her hands. She was so proud of Michael. We signed the necessary papers and back to Florida they went. Michael and I went on with our lives.

After our first child, we wanted another one, but, for some reason I couldn't get pregnant. Finally, we succeeded and our second son was born on January 6, 1979.

Little did we know that in the coming years our lives were about to be changed. Our happy family and our happy marriage would be severely tested. A disease most perplexing to man was going to sweep down upon us. I would become the victim of a major a illness—Manic Depression.

3

In January of 1979, I had just turned 30. After my pregnancy leave I returned to work. I couldn't have been happier. I had a husband and two healthy, beautiful sons. I was really on an up! My life had taken direction until May rolled around.

In May of 1979, I didn't feel well and Michael thought I should make an appointment to visit our family doctor. Across his office was the local funeral home. While waiting, I just kept focusing across the street and, in my mind, I felt I was going to die. I thought I had a physical problem, and, if not diagnosed soon I'd be gone. One physical symptom was chest pains, and in my mind thought I would have, or was having, a heart attack. I also had severe leg pains, which I thought indicated a blood clot, and a constant stomach ache, which I was sure, was a bleeding ulcer. I told the doctor of my physical symptoms. He checked me over and said, "It's your head. You are suffering from depression." I immediately went into a rage and told him there was nothing wrong with my brain. He didn't like my reaction, but, he gave me a prescription and sent me home. On my way out, I looked over at the funeral home, and, my thoughts turned to my brother. After all, it was there that I last saw him. All I could focus on was the fact that Michael would be raising our two boys on his own. I looked up into the clouds and told my brother that I would soon be with him. This was it. I knew I was dying. I was becoming very desperate and paranoid. I looked at the prescription and immediately bought a PDR (Physician's Desk Reference) to see what he had prescribed. It was an anti-depressant so, of course, the prescription went right into the trash.

I withdrew more as each day passed. I didn't feel safe knowing that, at any moment, the black cloud of death was going sweep down upon me. I didn't feel safe in the house or alone, but didn't want anyone around me either. Not feeling safe inside, I stayed outside most of the time. Michael worked days, the children were staying with his mother, and, I was alone. The reason I had to be outside was that, in my mind, I knew I was going to die. I wanted to be outside when death came so someone would notice and immediately call the Mogadore paramedics.

I didn't want to die inside the house, afraid that Michael would pick up the boys and come in the house to find me dead. I felt that this would be too traumatic on him and the children, so I would go outside every morning when Michael left for work and would not come in until he arrived home. I was completely paranoid.

Michael started to sense something was very wrong. He pleaded with me to go back to our family doctor or, at least, try the medication he had prescribed. I refused, telling him there was nothing wrong with my brain. That it was a physical problem. I flat out told him I knew I was going to die. At this point, I made him see our family attorney to have a will made out. He agreed to this just to make me happy. I didn't want to die without a will. It was a very important issue to me. After the will was made out and signed by us both, Michael definitely knew I needed help now. He made a phone call to Florida and talked at great length with my mother. He told me she was going to take the first flight out the next morning to come home and be with me. He had already talked to his family. Somehow, some way, he was going to get me help. I had gotten to the point where I couldn't even function.

Upon seeing my mother, I will never forget that look in her eyes. I had seen it before. She knew I was going to die, at least that was the impression in my sick mind. She had come from Florida to be with me when the time came.

Michael, his parents and my mother had gotten together. They knew it was useless to try and pursue it any further with our family doctor. For, at the mention of his name, I would become panic stricken. A plan had to be put into action.

It was on May 23, 1979, that Michael approached me about my gynecologist. My youngest child was five months old and Michael knew I had complete trust and faith in this fine young doctor. He had taken good care of me throughout the years, and, I had a good rapport with him. Michael wanted to call him and I thought it would be a great idea. After all, this man had a belief in me. After talking with my doctor at great length, Michael explained that my gynecologist would like me to go to the local hospital and be admitted. I felt that since my mother was here, Michael and my children would be taken care of, so I said I would go.

I was really ill and the ride to the hospital seemed like it took forever. I had to go through admitting, signing all sorts of forms which I didn't even bother to read. I just figured they were for insurance purposes, and, I was really too sick to care. Little did I know that I had actually signed myself into the psychiatric unit.

I knew I would be in good hands with my gynecologist so after signing the forms, an aide arrived to take me to the obstetrical floor. At least, that is where I thought I was going.

We went into a wing of the hospital I had never seen before. The aide opened a locked door and we were let in. When the door closed, I noticed it was locked. The hallway was covered with carpet and the rooms had regular beds in them. At the end of the hall was a room full of tables where men and women of all ages we sitting. All were dressed in casual clothing. Getting really paranoid over the whole situation, I asked to see my gynecologist. Michael tried to explain that he and my gynecologist both agreed I was probably suffering from post-partum depression. I wanted to see my gynecologist, and, I wanted to see him now. Devastation and anger set in.

How could my family knowingly let me sign myself into a psychiatric ward? My gynecologist was paged to the floor because I went completely out of control. How could he trick me? How could he even think that there was something wrong with my brain? He tried to explain that he didn't deal in depression. He felt I was suffering from post-partum depression since my last son was born in January. I was given a psychiatrist that was on duty at the time. I was informed that I would see my psychiatrist the next day. I had never met a shrink in my life, and, I didn't feel this was the right time to start. He came in and sat down, and, I immediately told him that, under no circumstances was I crazy. I had physical problems, and, once they were diagnosed and taken care of I would be back to my normal self. He informed me that I was suffering from depression. The words flew back and forth. I didn't care for him and he knew it.

I was assigned a primary nurse and a secondary nurse. Both were young, like me, and both seemed quite nice. I told both of them I didn't need to be in this type of ward. I had serious physical problems. They were to be in charge of keeping a chart on my daily activity and the things I would say, so that when my shrink arrived, he could easily breeze over their notes.

The only testing I had at this time was the usual, upon admission, except for an EEG, which is where they wire you, check your brain waves. It didn't hurt physically, but, it hurt emotionally to think that everyone thought my head was out of whack.

In my room there were metal lockers to put your clothing in. I hadn't even unpacked. I was so mad I walked over to the lockers and started beating on them, as if I had no sense left whatsoever. I beat them so hard that blood was coming out of my hand. My hand swelled up, and, when the nurses heard the pounding they came rushing down to see what the problem was. I felt no physical pain, but, the emotional pain was more than I could handle. I was immediately sedated and placed in a small room. The room I was placed in was a quiet area with a mattress on the floor. There was a TV camera which was linked up to the nurse's station.

It is used when a patient goes out of control so they don't hurt themselves, or, anyone else for that matter. After I settled down, my primary nurse came into the quiet area. I explained to her that I was sick, not mentally but physically. I told her the doctor would not run any of the tests to prove I was right. This nurse had a great belief in me and I knew, in my heart, she was going to help, but, I did not know when.

A psychiatric ward is completely different from any other part of a hospital. Every day you are expected to get up, make your bed, take a shower, and get ready for breakfast. They try to keep you in a daily routine. After breakfast, the doctors usually make their rounds. That was the worst part for me, because I did not want anything to do with this doctor. Every day, after he would leave, I would get into a fight with my locker. It was becoming a daily thing. One day my psychiatrist came in and I told him that if I was suffering from post-partum depression, I did not want any more children. I never wanted to feel this bad again, and, I demanded that he call my gynecologist and make the necessary arrangements to have my tubes tied. Knowing that Michael had had a vasectomy, he didn't see any point in my having the surgery. I insisted, and he actually said to me," Do you want your tubes tied so you can go out and whore around?" By that time I was in a state of rage. How dare he talk to me this way? I told him I had two healthy children and I didn't want to go through this again. He did call my gynecologist and the surgery was scheduled. After I had the surgery, he said to me, "Now you can go out and whore around all you want." This doctor and I were just not compatible.

We were allowed visitors twice a day, once in the morning and once in the evening. One day, my older sister showed up. During the course of the conversation, the subject of my five month old son came up. She informed me that I would never be mentally fit to take care of him and wanted my viewpoint on her and her husband adopting him. I couldn't believe what I was hearing. I went completely out of control.

She was asked to leave, and, I went wild. My room was a complete disaster. My hand was already swollen from past episodes, but, I beat and beat those lockers. I felt no pain, but, my hand was in bad shape. It was sedation time and back to X-ray. This time, not only did they X-ray my hand, but, they X-rayed my whole arm and shoulder area. I had actually left dents in the lockers. On returning from X-ray I was placed in the quiet area where my primary nurse came in and talked to me. She asked me what had gotten me so upset. I told her what my sister wanted. My sons were mine, not hers, and what gave her the right to even ask for one.

It was Sunday, and, the first time I would be able to visit my children. I knew the visit would be extremely difficult. I worried about my oldest son who was only four at the time. He and I were very close. I talked to the primary nurse and she said she would stick right by me. I was sitting at the table when visiting hours started. The door opened and people started coming in. I saw Michael and boys, and, the nurse assured me things would be fine. I knew different. My oldest caught a glimpse of me and started running up the hallway. He ran so fast and so hard he almost knocked the other visitors down. He finally reached me and jumped into my arm said, "Mommy, tell me where it hurts and I'll kiss it and make better." It was a very emotional situation. My primary nurse's and I were in tears. I picked him up and remember saying to him "You can't kiss this and make it well. It's something that you can't see.

It's not like the boo boos you get that I make feel better." He wanted me home, and, the entire nursing staff was in tears. My other son was so little all he could do was smile. He didn't know the pain I was experiencing.

My primary nurse said she would go to bat for me sooner or later. Sooner would have been better than later at this point. She asked me to try and cooperate. I had a real belief in her so I tried. One day my primary nurse didn't show up for work and I was given another nurse. She came in my room and sat down. She talked to me for a long time and brought up the subject of my brother. I totally lost it. My brother had meant so much to me that, when he died, I went to pieces. I found she had lost her brother too, from an auto accident. We both ended up in tears just holding each other. Finally, after 23 years of silence, the grief was pouring out. I so desperately wanted him back. We also discussed my feelings on the abortion. I could not shake the guilt I felt. It was overwhelming. They thought it might be best for a priest to come in and see me. I had told one nurse I had been to confession and was already forgiven, but the guilt was still there. A priest did show up and came in to talk to me. He offered me communion, and, we talked about the abortion. He told me over and over again that God was forgiving.

Every time I hear of someone who desperately wants children and cannot have them, I just feel terrible. I reflect back to abortion. I had extensive therapy in the hospital about how I felt, but to this day I still have guilt-ridden feelings. I just cannot forgive myself, and, I don't think I ever will.

It was time to engage in occupational therapy. A trained occupational therapist is in charge of getting patients busy with crafts, outdoor activities, picnics, and long walks to get the patient motivated. In therapy, I decided to make a belt for Michael. I am not a craft-oriented person. The only craft people in my family were my two sisters. I felt I had to make this belt, but, having little patience it took me a long time to complete it. I gave it to Michael and he was thrilled. Even to this day he wears it. I felt if I could make Michael a belt I could suffer through one more because I wanted one for myself. I finally got my belt together, but, it took some doing. I was about to run out of what little patience I had left.

During my stay, while I was under control, I got privileges. I got to go outside during evening visiting hours as long as Michael was there. This way I also got to see my children more often.

Eventually, the doctor figured I should try a home pass. This is when you are allowed out of the hospital for a short period to spend time with your loved ones in the surroundings that you had left. It's really hard being in the hospital and then trying to go back to a neighborhood after being gone so long. Michael had a surprise in store for me although I didn't know it at the time. Being a small town, I knew that when I got out of the car the neighbors would be watching. I could tell by watching them that they knew I had been in a psychiatric ward. I had wanted a new kitchen floor, and, as I walked in the house I saw that Michael and his uncle had torn up the old one and put down a new one. Needless to say, I was quite pleased. It made the kitchen seem so different.

The next day was going to be important, but, I did not know it. I was talking with my primary nurse when my doctor arrived. He left the room and the nurse walked right out behind him. She explained to him that she felt he should check my physical symptoms. He really got indignant with her. I heard her pleading with him to no avail. She came back in my room and said that she had tried, but, he wasn't about to listen to her.

During my stay, and feeling better from time to time, I did notice another psychiatrist walking around the unit. He always had interns with him and every-one just raved about how good he was. I also noticed that all of his patients were getting better, and, to be truthful I was feeling better, but, I was still sick. I kept a close eye on this doctor and he seemed to keep a close watch on me. It was really quite strange. One day I saw him walk into a private office where family members met with the staff. I noticed that there was no one else in the room. I had a chance and I felt now was the time to make my move. Filled with despair I walked quietly over to the door. Was it locked? I really didn't know. All I knew was I had to talk with him. I turned the handle and felt no resistance. Being des-perate I pushed my way in and shut it. I pleaded with this doctor to help me. I explained how long I had been there, and, I just knew he would be the one to make me feel better. He explained that he had been watching me for the past two months. He had even read my chart, but, hospital policy was that I couldn't switch to another doctor while under the care of one. He did say that he knew I was sick, and, that he would be willing to help me when I got released.

4

Well, my mother had to return to Florida. She had been here quite a while, and, my dad wanted her back home. In the meantime I told Michael about this doctor. At this point in time I was starting feel like my old self again, but, I knew deep down I was still physically sick. Michael promised to take me over to the new doctor upon my release. Shortly thereafter I was released from the hospital and returned home.

Time had passed and now we were getting into August. I felt like my old self again. I decided I didn't need to see another doctor. By October, I started feeling bad again, so Michael did make arrangements for me to see the psychiatrist that I so desperately wanted to see in the hospital. It was there in my psychiatrist office that I met Dr. Richard Shurrel, a psychologist. I talked with them at great length. The doctor suggested that I go back in the hospital for extensive testing. I knew that mentally I was better, but, physically I still felt the same. So here I was again in Admitting, signing the same papers I signed before. This time I knew what I was signing for. I knew I was going back to the psychiatric unit. I knew I was sick, and, I knew that this doctor was going to help me. At that moment, that was all that mattered.

I took a great liking to my new doctor. He didn't say much but, you could tell he was constantly thinking. He came in to see me and, I explained my physical symptoms which he had already read. He said very little and walked out. I thought it was strange, but somehow I knew he would help me. The next day I was scheduled for testing. He was thorough, and, I think I had every test the hospital had to offer. He told me that he had called an internal medicine doctor, the best in the field, to come and look at me. It was days before all the tests were run and the results were available. I was on very little medication as my new doctor had made some changes. Some days I felt some despair, and, on other days I felt great. The internist just like my psychiatrist had promised and checked me over. He too wanted to run tests. He ordered a massive blood study, and indeed it was massive. I had 24 tubes of blood drawn.

I really liked both of these doctors. I felt as if I was finally getting somewhere. One day, the internist showed up and sat down, chart in hand, and explained that my blood work was back and he wanted to go over his findings. He told me that I had a severe vitamin deficiency. I was lacking vitamins B6, B12, and Folic Acid. He also explained that the pain I was experiencing in my legs was due to an inflammation of the nerves in my legs. You see, it wasn't in my head. Next, he explained to me that my chest was hurting because I had a micro valve prolapse. I thought I was going to have a heart attack. But no, the valve flaps when under extreme stress, and the flapping was causing the pain. He immediately ordered a beta blocker that would take care of the pain.

I hadn't seen my psychiatrist all day which was quite unusual. I went to bed that night, and, around midnight he decided to make his rounds. He explained to me that the pain I was experiencing in my stomach was due to gall stones. He had consulted with a surgeon and they both felt that my gall bladder needed removed. It certainly was a great feeling to have faith in a doctor who followed up on the physical symptoms I was experiencing.

The surgeon came in and talked with me explaining the surgery. The primary nurse I had before in the ward had left. She wanted out of that line of work to try surgery. The surgeon knew I was scared. After all this was major surgery. I explained to him that the primary nurse I'd had before when I was in the unit was now on the surgical floor. The only way I would do the operation was if she could assist. He assured me he would see what he could do.

The psychiatric staff was to get me ready for surgery. I would leave the floor, go to surgery, recovery, and stay on the surgical floor for about a week. Michael and his mother arrived and off to surgery I went. I kept looking around for the primary nurse that had taken care of me on my first visit. Being drugged and everyone in green and wearing masks and hats, I couldn't see her. The doctor arrived and talked to me. I flat out told him there would be no operation without the nurse I had grown so close to and trusted so much. Being drugged I didn't realize she was there. She came over and pulled down her mask. Her smile lit up the whole room. Yes, I did feel safe. I was put to sleep, and, when I awoke she was right by my side in recovery. I told her, "See, it wasn't in my head." She bent down and hugged me and told me she believed me the whole time, and how sorry she was that she couldn't get the first doctor to listen. I remember her asking how Mike and the boys were, and, then she had to leave. When I awoke again I was on the surgical floor in a hospital bed, and, Michael was right there with me. He brought the children in on Sunday, and, I showed my oldest the gallstones that the doctor had removed. All he could say was, "Mommy why did you eat those stones?" At four years of age he just didn't understand. He didn't like the IV or the tube down my throat. They scared him. But, he wanted to take my gallstones home right away and show them to his friends.

My psychiatrist stopped in daily to see me and it was time, he said, to go back to the psychiatric floor. I explained to him I didn't feel I really needed to be there, but, for some reason, he assured me it was the right decision. He also said, "I believed in you. Now you must believe in me." Well, of course, I said I did and he said "Good. You need to be transferred back to the psychiatric unit." I did go, but, I sure wasn't happy about it. He wanted me to see a psychologist in the hospital and go through extensive testing. Also, he mentioned he was putting me on a different drug called Lithium. He explained that this drug was used for people suffering from mood swings. In order for the drug to work it had to reach a certain blood level, which takes time. He wanted to see how I reacted on it. I tried to tell him I felt great but, he insisted I take this drug.

I saw the psychologist in the hospital. He did extensive testing and made me look at ink blots, and, we did a lot of talking. It was him mostly asking questions and listening to my replies. He walked me back to the ward nearly three hours later. My room just happened to be by the nurses' station, and, the head nurse asked him how I made out. He didn't realize I was listening. I remember him saying "It's going to take years upon years of extensive therapy." Looking down the hall I caught a glimpse of my husband and my psychiatrist who stopped and chatted with the psychologist for quite a while. Afterwards, he stopped in to talk to Michael and me. He told us I was not suffering from post-partum depression. He explained to Michael that he wanted to get me on Social Security Disability due to the fact that I was suffering from Manic Depressive Psychosis, and had Erratic and Explosive Personality Disorder. It was his sincere feeling and, the feeling of the staff psychologist that I would never be able to return to work. He also explained that I would be going through more extensive psychological testing by another psychiatrist assigned by Social Security. He explained that the testing would be set up by the Social Security Administration. He also explained that, upon my release from the hospital, Dr. Rick Shurrel, the psychologist, would be taking care of my therapy. He would be monitoring my blood and medication management He said in very simple terms that, behaviorally, I was a classic example.

5

How do you come to grips knowing that you have a major mental illness and a real mental health problem? How was my family going to handle it, let alone my friends? I couldn't even grasp it. I was stunned.

Michael had told the doctor, through consultation, that I had walked into a neighborhood bank, and, without his knowledge borrowed $2500 on my own signature and had nothing to show for it. He brought up the fact that I had a love for automobiles, and, on several occasions, he would come home from work and find a new one sitting in the yard. I was working seven days a week, with little or no sleep, and, every charge card we owned was over its maximum limit. Michael also explained that on several occasions, when we planned a vacation, we would pack the car, and at the last moment I wanted to fly. Sometimes the vacations weren't even planned. I would call him at work and tell him to take a week off because I wanted to go away. Michael also told him that while I was in the hospital, these bills arrived, but knowing I was so sick he hadn't wanted to bring them up. The doctor explained to him that what I did were classic examples of Manic Depression. I had been on a manic high, spent money which we didn't have, and made irrational decisions. What goes up must come down, and I went into a severe depression. Michael's uncle came to our financial aid. Cars were traded between families and the bills were paid. Although Michael did pay his uncle back in full, if it weren't for him, we would have gone bankrupt.

I was always a happy-go-lucky type person. At least, I thought I was. I did a lot of strange things, but, I knew in my heart I wasn't a Manic Depressive. I finally returned home, and, it felt as if I had been gone forever. I visited the psychologist just to make Michael happy.

The psychiatrist was right. Social Security did call, and I went to see another psychiatrist. After talking with her, Social Security set up extensive testing with a group of psychologists in the area. The testing was intense. I talked to several different psychologist, looked at more ink blots, put pins in holes, and answered at least 1,000 questions. The testing took a total of five hours, non stop. Not being a patient person I wanted to know right then and there what the results were. I was informed that a rehabilitation agency would be contacting me.

I don't remember exactly how long it was, but, I got the call to go in to talk to a counselor. Personally, I didn't think I needed rehabilitation. I felt great. Michael and I walked in and sat down, and, the woman in charge had my test results from the hospital and Social Security. This woman with a vanilla folder had all the information that I wanted to know. She looked it over, looked at me, and said "You are so severely disabled you will never work again. I am placing your folder in our 'DEAD FILE.'" She explained to Michael that I was, indeed, eligible and would be receiving Social Security based my earnings and for my two children. She also told him that the checks would come in his name, not mine. We walked out and got in the car. For once in my life, I couldn't say a thing. How could this be? I worked for a major rubber company in which I was ready to move up. How could I ever face my friends and family? How was I going to tell my children? How would I tell my boss I would never be coming back to work? I had no answers to any of these questions.

Everyone was saying I had a major mental illness and I would never work again. I was devastated. I was due for a blood test, after which I knew I would prove to everyone the diagnosis was wrong. I went off the Lithium.

6

I did test the diagnosis, my moods started to swing, and I started to drink. All the drinking did was control the mania to a certain degree. I became agitated very easily. Some nights, I couldn'1 fall asleep. I became so agitated that I ended up destroying over $2,000 worth of furniture and a $500 reel to reel tape recorder. I threw anything and everything I got my hands on. I even lashed out Michael. Michael immediately called the doctor, and I ended up back in the hospital. The doctor asked me why in the hell I ever went off the Lithium. I flat out told him I couldn't believe I had a major illness, and, I was going to prove it.

This time, I spent approximately three weeks in the hospital getting my blood level up to acceptable limits. This was also t time my father came to visit me. He said, "Let's get the hell out of here." So I used a four-hour pass I had gotten. My dad took me out to get something to eat and blamed the whole situation on the drugs I had taken when I was younger. He said that if Michael had any brains he would divorce me. He wanted to know how in the hell one of his daughters could ever end up with a mental illness. He felt everything I had ever done was done wrong. It was a really nice visit, if you happen to be a person who likes being put down.

If testing the diagnosis didn't almost ruin my marriage, being more on the manic side of the illness almost did. When you are manic you don't think your thoughts are really distorted. Even on Lithium I was able to go manic to a degree. During one high, I went out and had an affair. I thought that was great, but, of course I wasn't think properly. When I came down and realized what I had done, I went to Michael and told him. This happened on more than one occasion.

Michael was at his wits end. After all, I had tested the doctor and now it was his turn. I was absolutely nasty to him, downright mean. I lashed out at him every chance I had. Michael was considering divorce and I really couldn't blame him. Of course my family agreed with him. He talked to a priest and my psychologist before deciding to take drastic measures. My psychologist explained to him that this was how life was going to be. He told Michael that he wouldn't blame him if he walked out. He had every reason in the world, and, no one would blame him. He also told Michael that even though things were bad and life didn't look promising, things might get better. Michael had to decide whether or not he loved me enough to weather out the storm. It was going to last a long time because there was, and is, no cure for Manic Depression. Michael said that he needed help in dealing with all the events that disrupt our lives. He too, would be in therapy learning how to deal with my illness. He loved me enough to stay and try to cope.

Feeling extremely guilty about what I had done, I didn't feel I was doing him or the children any good. My father was right. I was a complete failure. I felt sorry for Michael and the children and the hell they were going through. I felt sorry for myself. I took a drug overdose, but, my suicide attempt failed. I woke up in the hospital and remember Michael asking me why I did it. I told him that he and the children would be better off without me. I couldn't live with the illness, and, I didn't think he should have to either. I felt no one understood or really cared. Through the years, I felt a sense of competition, being the middle child. I didn't want to compete or be compared to anyone anymore. I remained hospitalized again, this timely for a short period of time. After my release, I started seeing my psychologist again.

7

A short time later my psychologist quit working for my psychiatrist. I was assigned a psychiatric nurse. I was really upset. I wanted my psychologist back, but, there was no way my psychiatrist would let me see him. If I went on my own to see him my insurance would not cover it because the psychiatrist did not order it. Eventually, he did concede, and wrote the necessary letter for me to see my psychologist again.

In 1983, after a tremendous bout with my older sister, I just couldn't handle it anymore. On impulse I went out and bought a gun. Filled with alcohol and drugs, and with only one bullet in the chamber, I retired to our rec room. Michael noticed something was definitely wrong. I felt bad and my mind was becoming sicker and sicker. I really didn't want to live anymore. Michael tried talking to me telling me there was nothing worth taking my life over. I continued to drink, and, he called the local police. At one point, Michael tried to grab the gun. He was fortunate it didn't go off. I didn't want to hurt him. Every police officer in the village was in the house. Everyone wanted to talk. I told them all the they didn't understand me or my sister. They called in an off-duty officer who had gone to school with my sister. He talked to me and understood my feelings about my sister. He graduated with her and knew what she was like. After all he had dated her at one time. He said that she wasn't worth this, and, he asked me to give him the gun. After time, I did allow him to take the gun. He understood.

My doctor was called immediately. It was customary in this type of case to go straight to a psychiatric hospital. My doctor explained to the police that, under no circumstances was I to be taken to a psychiatric hospital. Instead, I was to be taken to the local hospital and placed back in the psychiatric ward. The police officer asked me if I would go. I didn't want to, of course, but, I was taken by cruiser to the local hospital anyway. He promised me he wouldn't leave until I got settled in. The officer went through the emergency room with me. My doctor had already called ahead for medication to be administered upon my arrival, and, I was placed in the psychiatric ward. I was back in the hospital again. My ups just kept going up until I would reach erratic behavior. So, along with the Lithium, I was given a major tranquilizer. To this date, that was my last hospitalization.

There have been a few times that I have almost ended up there, but, it has been avoided by quick action on Michael's part.

8

How was Michael going to curb my spending sprees? What was he to do with a compulsive shopper? I can't speak for everyone, but I can tell you what happened to me. All my charge accounts were closed and the plates destroyed. Michael opened another checking account in his name only. We still have our joint checking, but, Michael watches closely how much money is in it. When it gets to a certain point, he transfers the funds. Our savings account is in both names, but, if I make a withdrawal over a certain amount the bank will phone Michael immediately. Because I have a love for automobiles, he took me out and told me exactly how much I could spend. I thought that was great until he put the vehicle in his name. In this way, I cannot trade it as I have done in the past.

Michael knows I'm not happy with no money in my pocket, so he allows me so much money per week. When it's gone, it's gone. When I go to my psychiatrist or psychologist the bill has to be paid right then. Having tremendous coverage we can coordinate benefits. But the bills are actually paid first by Michael. When the checks arrive, one will come in my name and the other in his name to cover the visit. If I decide to cash mine and not send it to the doctor, which pays for my visit, it comes out of my allowance. So I endorse the checks. In this way, the visit is already paid for before I even get there. I surely don't want it coming out of my pocket.

When it comes to charities, Michael steps in. He decides when to give, and how much. When it comes to gift giving Michael will, at Christmas, sit down and write the names of the people to whom we wish to give a gift. By each persons name there is an allotted amount. When buying clothing for myself, Michael accompanies me. He isn't cheap, but, he's not a spend thrift either. He buys me what I need when I need it. My personal viewpoint on this situation is I don't like it, of course. Michael has been able to establish a moderate, but adequate, savings which he won't dip into unless it is a real emergency. Through his payroll savings plan at work, the account grows and grows. Sometimes when I look at it, my mind goes into overdrive. But I know I can't touch it. Michael allows so much for groceries, but, then again, I have a real phobia about the grocery store and the major malls. I write down what we need from the store and Michael takes the boys and does the shopping. I have a complete panic attack in the grocery store. To this day, I have not been able to overcome it. If there is any grocery money left, it is set aside. We use it if we need to pick up bread or milk during the week, or for our trips to the meat market or an outlet store nearby.

It has been hard to get accustomed to, but, Michael has complete control over my spending. In the past, I have spent and spent, never having anything to show for it. I bought automobiles and gotten tired of them two weeks later. The longest I have ever owned a vehicle is the one I have now. It's only two years old. My mother used to say, "When it gets dirty, it's time to trade it in." She also used to say, "Put your money in the bank. They aren't going to steal it from you."

I used to love to drink, but drinking doesn't mix with my medication. After too many drinks, I get completely out of control. It's a proven fact that every time I drink, I end up in the hospital. Both of our families drink and, on special occasions and during the holidays, it is especially hard for me. I want to drink but Michael knows what happens, so we usually end up leaving early. There is a wine we found through a psychiatric nurse that has no alcohol content at all, none whatsoever. But, I was never much of a wine drinker. Now it's Diet 7-Up. Things change. They have to order for me to keep on an even keel.

I am still quite vulnerable to stress and self-destructiveness. To vent these frustrations, Michael purchased a 15 speed bike for me. He thought I would soon give up riding, but I haven't. I ride and ride until I wear myself out. In the winter I ride an exercise bike. He also bought me a tape of Jane Fonda, and I exercise to her on our VCR. Stress can get me even though I exercise.

9

I do have some strange phobias. I feel very safe and secure with Michael. I can even manage the grocery store with him by my side if it is one that is open 24 hours a day, and we go around three in the morning. This year, for the first time I went to a benefit. It was tough. On the way there I began to get panic stricken, but, with Michael at my side I managed. When I become panic stricken, I feel as if I'm going to die. My hands, feet, and forehead start to sweat. I get a feeling of dizziness, and a faint feeling overcomes me.

Another phobia I have is going on vacation. When I was younger, I had the opportunity to visit every state except Alaska and Hawaii. Now, I don't feel safe outside the state. If something were to happen, I want my doctors close at hand. Even when I ride my bike, I carry my medical card with my doctor's name on it. All the medications I'm on, and an EKG is on the back of the card. I always carry it. It takes a lot for me to have trust in a doctor. It really does. I'm not the only person my doctor gives a medical card to. He gives them to all his patients. I have the security of knowing that if I am by myself and have a panic attack and pass out, they will able to contact him and Michael. Michael and my doctors represent my security.

Sometimes I know I should call the doctor but, being the type of person I am, I don't. Michael calls and they know there is trouble brewing. His phone call is returned immediately. My psychologist has given us his home phone number, and, Michael carries it with him at all times. When I have an episode, I feel sooner or later, I will get over it. Michael sizes up the situation and decides whether I need immediate attention, or if I just need an appointment as soon as possible.

I have a great rapport with my psychologist. I have been with him since 1979, and, he has counseled Michael and the children throughout the years. I admit, there have been times when I have walked out of a session with him because of my anger. Sometimes he can get me to come back in and sometimes he can't. If he can't, he usually calls me at home and I meet with him again after I have calmed down. He tries to lead me in the right direction, and tells me when I am heading for trouble. He is also teaching me that, since I am manic, people can't always act on my ideas. It is quite frustrating to me, but, at the same time I don't realize I am stressing people out. We have really been working hard on this. I would never intentionally stress someone out. I just don't realize I am doing it unless it's pointed out to me.

When my family heard the results of diagnosis, they were devastated. They, of course, didn't want to believe it. They told me I should definitely not tell anyone. They really backed away from me. They were scared. They didn't understand or want the knowledge or the education that was readily available to them. My mom was different. She wanted the knowledge, and truly tried to understand the illness. She explained it to my two sisters. On various occasions, they had experienced my explosive behavior, since it had been directed at them. I never hit them, but, I scared them. At times, I've tried to say I'm sorry, but, the damage had been done. Half of the time I didn't even remember what I exploded about.

The family got together when my parents came from Florida for a visit, but, it was really different. My mother was the glue that kept my sisters and me on neutral ground. She would listen to me and try to explain to them why I was so upset. In October of 1983, my mother was diagnosed as having cancer. The cancer was so bad, I was heartsick. When my brother died of cancer at the age of 14, it tore me up. Now my mother, the only one that truly wanted to understand me, was dying.

Upon hearing this sad news, I knew that she was to be operated on immediately. I couldn't bring myself to get on a plane to be with her. Emotionally, it took its toll. She had less than 50% chance of making it through surgery. My older sister flew to Florida to be with my father. My mother survived the operation, but wasn't expected to live long. My sister called me and explained that if I didn't come to Florida, I would have to live with the guilt the rest of my life. My mother had always been there for me, but, I just couldn't get on that plane. I had the ticket in my hand, but, my feet were like cement implanted in the ground. My mother wasn't up to traveling, but in March of 1984 she knew she had to come here. Her doctor objected because she was so weak, but she managed to get on the plane. She came because she felt the need to talk to me. When she arrived, I started crying. She had to be helped out of car and held up. She was once a strong and independent person. It was heartbreaking to see her this way. We sat one night and she told me she wasn't going to live much longer. She said she knew I didn't want to hear it, but it was true. She explained that my dad had been good to her through the 45 years they had been married, and, that all through her sickness he had taken the best possible care of her. He had learned to cook and clean and made sure she was well cared for. She explained that, being so close through the years and doing almost everything together, he would never be able live alone after her death. She knew that, eventually, he would want to remarry. I told her I could never accept anyone else, or call any other woman 'mom.' She told me I didn't have to call anyone else 'mom'. I didn't even have to like the person, just show respect for whoever it was he chose to live out his remaining days with. I sat and listened with my insides crumbling. I believed there would be a miracle and she would live. It just had to be that way. At this point in my life, my visits to the doctor went from once every two weeks to almost twice a week. I just couldn't deal with the thought of losing my mother. She told me she knew I had good intentions of coming to see her, but, she also knew why I couldn't get on that plane. She pleaded with me not to feel guilty about it. She also promised that, God willing, she would come back in and visit me. But she was so thin and weak, I thought I would never see her again. Her main concern was my health, not hers. She came back in May just like she promised. By that time, her stomach had become greatly extended. She was ordered by her doctor to see a cancer specialist here, while on vacation, for blood work. While here, she visited with her closest friend. I didn't know this at the time, but she explained her concern over what might happen to me when she died.

When my mother left, we both knew we would never see each other again. I made a call to the doctor that my mother visited while here in town. She told me my mother was very sick and to get prepared because she was dying. She told me my mother had three months to live, at the most. That would be June to August. The doctor was right. She passed away in September. My sisters approached me again saying I should be in Florida with my mother. I went down the street to my mother's best friend and told her I just couldn't go. We would purchase airplane tickets, and, the day before I was prepared to leave I would panic, and I mean panic. She told me it didn't matter what anyone said. She and my mom had had a long talk in May, and my mother understood. My mother had admitted to her that she would have loved for me to come, but not if it was going to put me back in the hospital. She knew the thought of her dying was doing a number on my head.

While my mother was here in May, she told me that she would be cremated because she wanted desperately to be buried by her only son. That was the only way it could be done. She knew my feeling on cremation. I didn't want mother put in a blazing furnace. She told me it would be fine and that it was truly what she wanted. I was crushed. I was being tortured by my sisters for not going to my mother's side, and I was torturing myself because I felt like a failure. After all my mother was always here for me. Every day, right up until the end, I called to talk with her. I remember her telling me that no matter what happened, she loved me.

On September 10, 1984, around 4:00 in the morning the dreaded call came. My father said, "Your mom is gone. I started crying and he said, "Don't cry. She's suffered enough. She's better off." My older sister got on the phone and said "You wouldn't be crying if you had come here and seen her. You'd be glad her suffering is over." I tried explaining that there was no way possible I could have made it there, and would she please try to understand. Well, she wasn't very understanding.

My mother was to have services in Florida and then be brought back here to be buried beside my brother with graveside services. As hard as it was, I made the arrangements for the service. Another phone call came from my sister in Florida. They now wanted the services in a funeral home so I retraced and made other arrangements. Another call, and they wanted to have church services. At that point, I was so devastated, I couldn't pick up the phone again. It was then my mother's best friend walked in. I started to tell her of the events that were taking place. My dad called and said "Okay, what do you want?" I said, "I want donations to be made in my mother's name to the Mental Health Association here in town." I certainly didn't want them to go to the Cancer Society because, in my mind, they had already gotten my brother and my mother. He said, "Fine." My mother's friend was still with me when the phone rang again. My older sister called me to say that, "…under no circumstances will donations be made in my mother's name to mental health. You are the only mental degenerate in the family, and, we certainly don't was anyone to think our mother died of a mental illness." Push came to shove and my mom's friend took the phone and asked them not to call, that emotionally, I was on the verge of collapse. As a good friend of my mothers, and being a registered nurse, she wanted me to come home with her. I hesitated, but went. She made me eat, gave me some pills to take, and had me lie down. I was on the verge of going into the hospital and, that was the last thing my mother would have wanted, and she knew it.

Having services in Florida and then arranging services here takes time. My mother died September 10th, but the services here in town weren't until September 19th. Nine days of complete torture.

My father arrived and started drinking, saying if there were truly a God then his son and his wife would still be here. He drank himself to the point where he started crying for my older sister who lived in Pennsylvania. She came running and began blaming me for getting dad so upset. The fact was that I had done nothing. Before the services, I did explode at my sisters. I came apart because I was emotionally sick. I knew my mother was to be cremated, but, my sister decided that urns did not look like my mother's taste. Her remains were put in a cookie jar and dropped off at the cemetery.

To this day, my older sister will have nothing to do with me. In fact, she doesn't want anyone like me around them. I admit, I did say some terrible things. I was sick, you see, and they don't believe in mental illness. They believe that a person should be strong enough to face things. I will never forget the services, because it was actually the last time I saw my two sisters until recently when my sister Becky came back into life.

Even to this day, Michael won't let me visit the cemetery, under orders from my psychologist. After my mother's death, I tried to dig up her remains. I was emotionally disturbed over the fact that her remains were put in a cookie jar and that her ashes weren't even blessed. When it comes time to put flowers on the grave, Michael makes a donation in my mother and brother's name to save me the emotional turmoil I would experience while in the cemetery.

I lost faith in God again and didn't attend Mass for almost a year. The boys started asking their father why, I wouldn't go to church. The night before mom died, the sermon was on Lazarus and how God promised that he would be brought back to life—a real miracle. After hearing that, and experiencing a thought disorder, I couldn't understand why he wouldn't bring my mother back. After almost a year, I talked to a friend and was inspired, so I decided to talk to a Priest. I told the Priest how I felt and he asked, "Would you want your mom back just so you could experience her death again?" I told him I wasn't able to handle it the first time, and I knew I couldn't handle it twice. August 10, 1985, on my mother's birthday, I returned to Mass. Deep inside, I knew it would the best present I could give her, Michael, or the boys. It had been eleven months since her death. We went to church again as a family.

10

Over the years, I have tried to call and talk to my family. However, they assured me of their feelings and that is that. The rejection I feel hurts. They call me a failure because I couldn't walk on that airplane to see my mother while she still lived. I know how they feel, and, I know how my father feels about mental health. I have been in therapy and know how they all feel. My psychologist wants me to keep the lines of communication open between my dad and me, even though they are strained.

My mother was right. My dad did remarry, one year after her death. I have talked with the woman on the phone, but have never met her. I understand from my father that she is great seamstress. One day I asked if she would do me a favor and she asked, "If I do it wrong, will you blow up at me?" After that remark, I knew she had heard from my father and had met my sisters and had probably already formed an opinion about me without ever having met me. That was a real shame because, in talking with her, I had never gotten out of line or said anything to her to give her any reason for that remark.

In extensive therapy on family rejection with my psychologist, he said that life has to go on and you cannot educate someone that doesn't want the education. I finally accepted how my family feels, and I have been living with the knowledge since then.

For six long years, I had the same psychiatrist. One day, he went on vacation and liked it so well he never came back. I was devastated. I really didn't know what I was going to do. Being hospitalized on several occasions, I'd met a lot of the psychiatrists. I knew which psychiatrist I liked and which one's I didn't like.

I have a really good friend and, knowing me as well as she does, she thought of a psychiatrist that I might like. She told me to call Dr. Mosteller. I called him, but he wasn't taking any new patients. Starting all over again was a big step to take. I really didn't feel I was up to it. I met the doctor and we sat down and the first thing he did was put me in the hospital for three days and take me off of lithium and change my medication. I knew he had psychologists on staff and that was the next order of business. Under no circumstances would I leave the one I had. My mind was made up. He was very kind and gentle and said he would handle my medication and that I could continue my therapy with Dr. Shurell, the psychologist I knew and trusted.

This year, I rode my bike 20 miles for a fund raiser. Sixteen miles out I got really sick and confused. At one point I didn't even know where I was. I managed to get back on track, knowing that Michael was only four miles away. I just needed enough strength to get to him. When I did, he knew I was in need of immediate medical attention. My internist was a 30 minute drive from where we were. My psychiatrist was only five minutes away. He was the closest, and that's where we headed. Upon arrival, he looked me over. I was in bad shape. Being an avid bike rider himself, he knew I was suffering from heat exhaustion. He had seen it before. He told me that, due to the fact that I don't sweat much, the heat builds up. He had seen many people have mini strokes while biking. He said it had scared me because my mind was trying to tell my body something and the two didn't connect. He told Michael to take me home and he would call me that night. Michael had to go to work. He didn't want to go, but, I told him to go ahead. After all, the doctor said I would be fine. I just needed rest. That night my psychiatrist called. He really did care! I came right off the street and into his office, without appointment and yet, he didn't charge me. I feel I'm in go hands with him. Since our talk, and since my ride, I truly believe this man has my best interest at heart. I thank God I decided to give him a chance because he is truly a fine doctor.

Dr. Mosteller, Christina's daughter Lisa, Mike and I rode 20 miles.

At a follow up meeting Dr. Mosteller diagnosed me being a type II diabetic and placed me on a treatment plan which included medication. The treatment worked and I no longer have a problem with the diabetes.

11

I have finally accepted my diagnosis. Sometimes I fall short and when I visit my psychologist or psychiatrist I will ask, "Do you really think I'm a Manic Depressive?" Everytime, they both answer, "most definitely." I feel the only reason I have been able to accept the diagnosis is because of my strong support system, my doctors, my friends, and especially Michael and the children.

I know there is no cure for Manic Depression. I suffer the mood swings. It truly isn't easy to accept not knowing from day to day how I am going to feel. I think the hardest part of all is the stigma attached to my illness. Michael and I both know that any minute, any day, any week, month, or year I could suffer a major relapse. I still have a tremendous problem where stress is concerned. I am quite vulnerable, and it tends to take its toll. I am happy to say I have not had any relapses the last twenty years.

I thank God I have Michael. What other man would stay and take the verbal and physical abuse I have put him through the past eight years. He seems to deal better with my illness than I do. He always has a word of encouragement.

When it would have been so easy for him to walk out that door, he stayed. Mental illness is a constant battle. Not only for the people who suffer from it, but for their families as well. I know I'm not alone. Millions of people suffer from mental health problems that require periodic psychiatric hospitalization. Years ago, if I had been diagnosed mentally ill, I would have ended up in an institution and probably left there till I died. I know the treatment of the mentally ill has changed dramatically over the years. We are fortunate to have a Mental Health Association in our community. People concentrating together trying to find solutions to problems, providing the best possible treatment to those who are afflicted.

Over the years, through out my illness, I have occasionally been able to volunteer my time in the fight against mental illness. My husband has been right by my side in all my endeavors. The Executive Director of the Mental Health Association and staff all know I suffer from Manic Depression. At times, they have undergone tremendous stress caused by the fundraising ideas that float around in my mind. Their main concern has never bee how much money I could raise, but for my health. These people are truly caring individuals and they gave me hope, encouragement, and selfworth when I had none left. They are mental health professionals fighting a never ending battle, not for me, but for anyone that suffers with an emotional disorder. There is a mental health bell that is the symbol of this organization. It carries the inscription, "CAST FROM THE SHACKLES WHICH BOUND THEM. THIS BELL SHALL RING OUT HOPE FOR THE MENTALLY ILL AND VICTORY OVER MENTAL ILLNESS."

I don't hide my illness in a closet any longer. If I can't accept it, how can I ever expect anyone else to. I am a Manic Depressive. I no longer suffer from an Erractic and Explosive Personality Disorder. I'm far from being cured and have several relapses. But, I still have hope. In my heart, I know that someday I'll hear that bell and victory will be mine. I pray for others who suffer from emotional disorders. I feel fortunate I have a mental health team that works with me, Michael, the boys, and our many friends support me.

Conclusion

I didn't write this for fame, fortune, or notoriety. I felt it had to be written, because there are books and articles about Manic Depression, but they have all been written by mental health professionals, not by a patient. This is a true account from my childhood on through the age of 30, when the chemical imbalance in my brain was diagnosed. It takes you through my bouts with alcohol and drugs, fears, phobias, deaths of loved ones, suicide attempts, family rejection, psychiatric admissions, and the mental health care I received. Most importantly, it tells you how a family has lived and the help they so desperately needed in order to deal with the Manic Depressive Psychosis.

My husband has been a true asset in helping me get this together, because there were many things that happened that I couldn't remember. He remembers because he lived through it all too. He reached out for the education and awareness that he and our children needed in order to deal with a wife and mother suffering a serious mental illness. Michael feels that living with me and my illness has made him more aware of the mental health problems that plague our society. He feels my mood swings bring excitement and the unknown into his life. Every day is different, so we definitely don't lead a dull existence.

Michael is a devout Catholic and he knows God won't send him any more than he can handle. We live day by day, with hope in our hearts and a prayer on our lips.

God Bless you Michael.

978-0-595-38285-9
0-595-38285-1